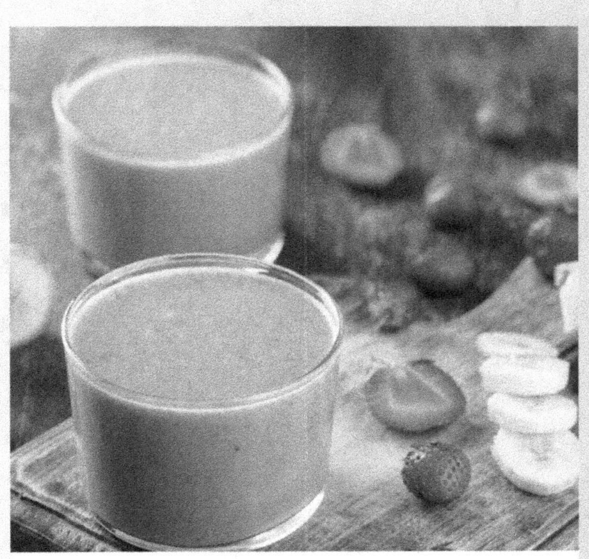

SMOOTHIES FOR WEIGHT GAIN

DR. MARGERY J. ENGLAND

Smoothie For Weight Gain

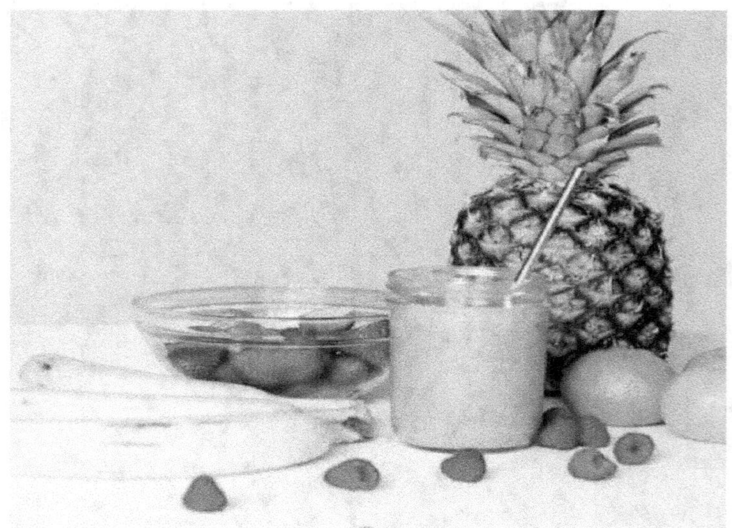

20 Wholesome, Healthy and Nutritious Smoothie Recipe For Weight Gain

Dr. Margery J. England

Copyright © 2023, Dr. Margery J. England

About The Author (Dr. Margery J. England)

Dr. Margery J. England expertly marries culinary artistry with scientific insight. A celebrated chef, she is also a leading authority on the wellness benefits of juices and smoothies. From world-class kitchens to rigorous academic research, Margery's passion is clear: crafting dishes and drinks that not only delight the senses but nourish the body.

This book captures her unique approach to blending flavor with function. Immerse yourself in her delicious wisdom and let your health—and taste buds—reap the benefits.

Today, Dr. England is celebrated for her innovative approach to integrating flavor with function. Her juices and smoothies are more than just beverages; they're carefully crafted elixirs that invigorate, heal, and energize. Her recipes embody her philosophy: that food should serve both our body's needs and our soul's desires.

Table Of Contents

Introduction

In a bustling city, Alex, a determined and spirited individual, struggled to gain weight and build a stronger physique. Despite countless efforts, she found a smoothie recipe book called "Smoothie For Weight Gain" that offered her a unique blend of recipes to nourish her body and soul. Alex decided to try the smoothie recipes gotten from the book. The first sip of the smoothie sparked a newfound energy and vitality within Alex, and they returned daily, transforming their bodies and spirit.

As Alex's transformation became apparent, confidence radiated from w ithin, and their once hesitant steps now strode with purpose and determination. The secret behind the transformative smoothie was the belief that even in the busiest cities, there was a hidden oasis of hope and nourishment. This story is about resilience, finding the right path amidst uncertainty, and discovering that sometimes the most potent elixirs are not just the ones we drink but the ones that awaken the strength within us.

Smoothie Recipes For Weight Gain

If you're looking to gain weight in a healthy and delicious way, smoothies can be an excellent option! Packed with nutrient-dense ingredients, these weight gain smoothies are perfect for anyone looking to add extra calories, protein, and healthy fats to their diet. Whether you're an athlete, a fitness enthusiast, or simply trying to build muscle, these 30 smoothie recipes will help you reach your weight gain goals. Get ready to blend and enjoy!

1. Classic Banana Peanut Butter Power

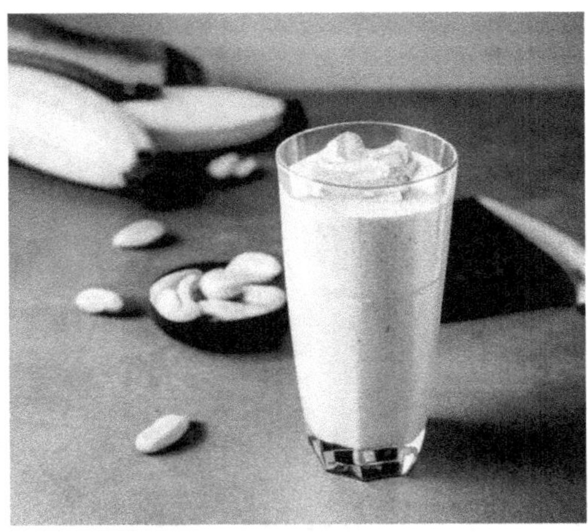

Ingredients:
- 2 ripe bananas
- 2 tablespoons natural peanut butter
- 1 cup whole milk
- 1 tablespoon honey
- 1/4 cup oats
- 1/2 teaspoon vanilla extract

Preparation:
1. Peel and chop the bananas.
2. Combine all ingredients in a blender.
3. Blend until smooth and creamy.

4. Pour into a glass and enjoy!

Prep Time: 5 minutes

2. Chocolate Avocado Dream

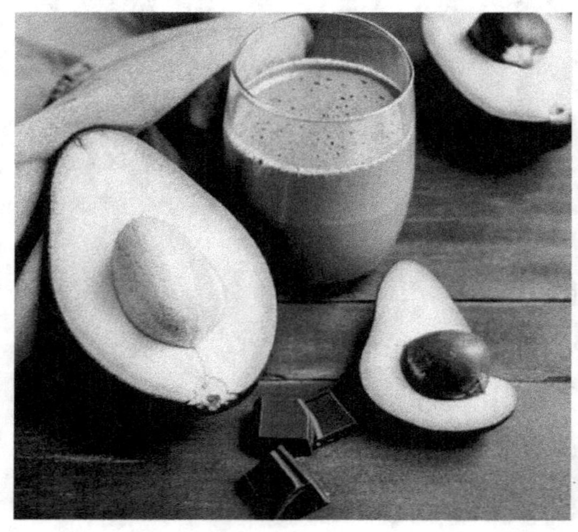

Ingredients:
- 1 ripe avocado
- 2 tablespoons cocoa powder
- 1 cup almond milk
- 2 tablespoons honey
- 1/4 cup Greek yogurt
- 1/2 teaspoon cinnamon

Preparation:

1. Scoop out the avocado flesh.
2. Combine all ingredients in a blender.
3. Blend until well mixed.
4. Pour into a glass and savor the chocolate goodness!

Prep Time: 5 minutes

3. Tropical Mango-Coconut Bliss

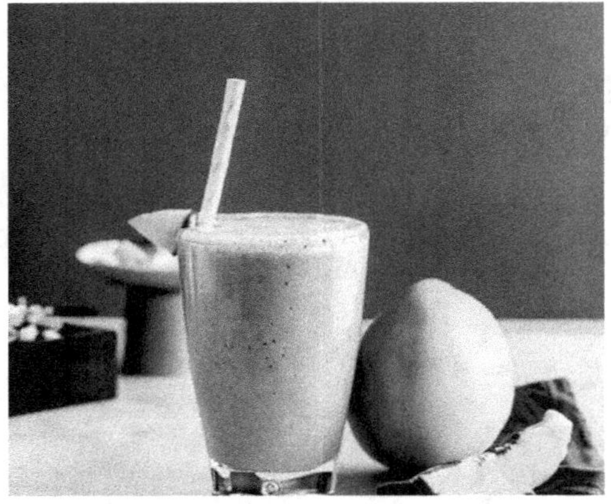

Ingredients:
- 1 cup frozen mango chunks
- 1/2 cup canned coconut milk

- 1/2 cup orange juice
- 1 tablespoon chia seeds
- 1 tablespoon shredded coconut

Preparation:

1. Combine all ingredients in a blender.

2. Blend until smooth and creamy.

3. Pour into a glass and imagine yourself on a tropical island!

Prep Time: 5 minutes

4. Berry Almond Powerhouse

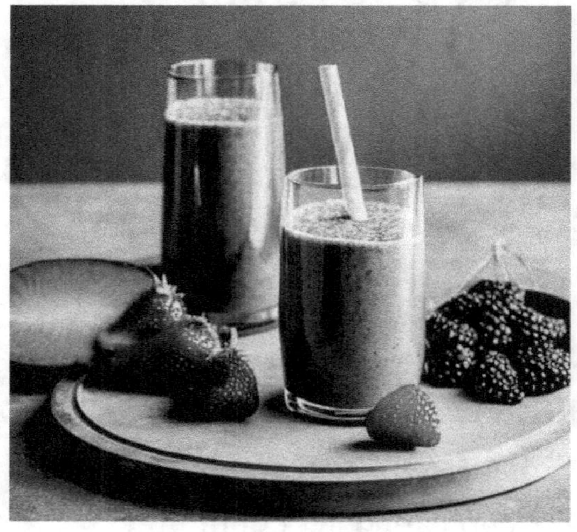

Ingredients:

- 1 cup mixed berries (strawberries, blueberries, raspberries)
- 1/4 cup almond butter
- 1 cup whole milk
- 1 tablespoon maple syrup
- 1/4 cup rolled oats

Preparation:

1. Wash the berries and remove stems.
2. Combine all ingredients in a blender.
3. Blend until well combined.
4. Pour into a glass and enjoy the burst of berry goodness!

Prep Time: 5 minutes

5. Nutty Chocolate-Banana Blast

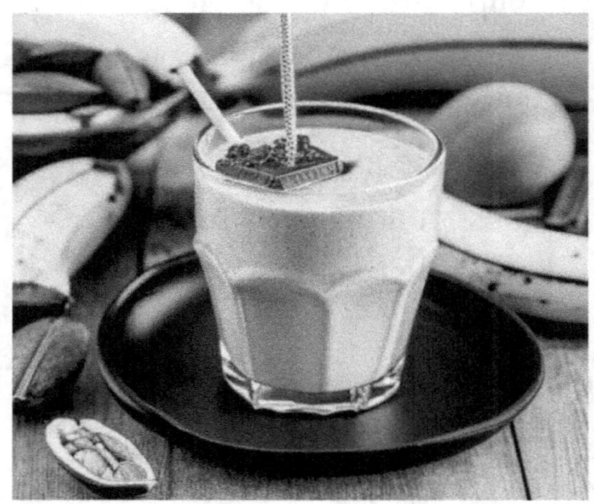

Ingredients:

- 1 ripe banana
- 2 tablespoons almond butter
- 1 cup chocolate almond milk
- 1 tablespoon cocoa powder
- 1 tablespoon honey
- 1/4 cup granola

Preparation:

1. Peel and chop the banana.
2. Combine all ingredients in a blender.
3. Blend until smooth and creamy.

4. Pour into a glass and relish the chocolate and banana combo!

Prep Time: 5 minutes

6. Spinach-Berry Power Punch

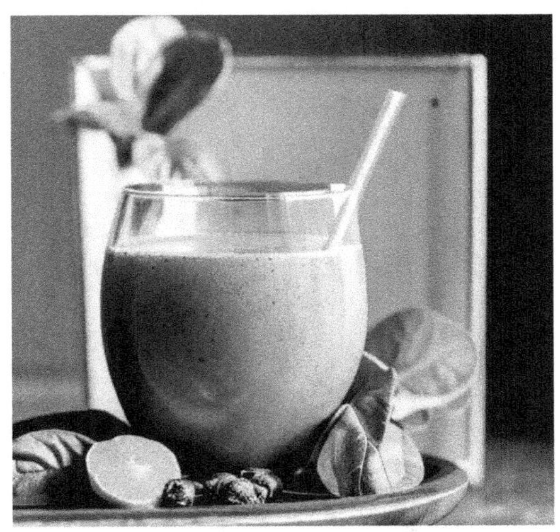

Ingredients:
- 1 cup fresh spinach leaves
- 1 cup mixed berries (strawberries, blueberries, blackberries)
- 1/2 cup Greek yogurt
- 1 tablespoon honey

- 1/2 cup water or coconut water

Preparation:

1. Wash the spinach leaves thoroughly.
2. Combine all ingredients in a blender.
3. Blend until well mixed.
4. Pour into a glass and enjoy a nutritious green smoothie!

Prep Time: 5 minutes

7. Creamy Vanilla-Date Delight

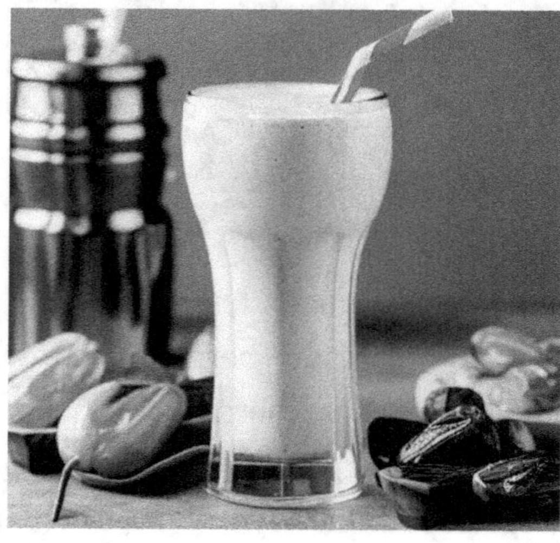

Ingredients:

- 2 ripe bananas
- 4 Medjool dates, pitted
- 1 cup whole milk
- 1 teaspoon vanilla extract
- 1/4 cup almonds

Preparation:

1. Peel and chop the bananas.
2. Combine all ingredients in a blender.
3. Blend until creamy and smooth.
4. Pour into a glass and experience the sweetness of dates!

Prep Time: 5 minutes

8. Cherry-Almond Protein Power

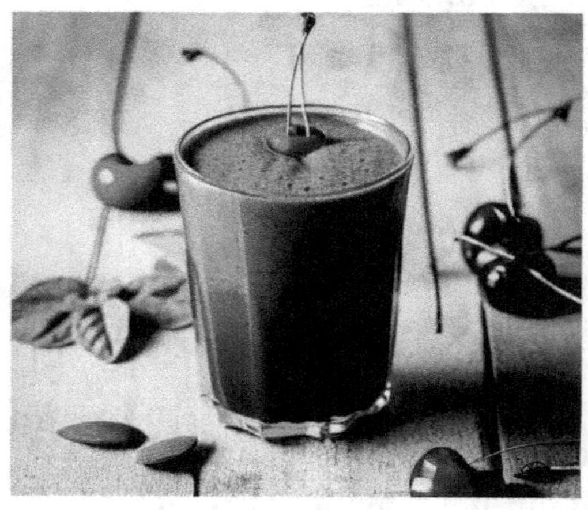

Ingredients:

- 1 cup frozen cherries
- 1/4 cup almond butter
- 1 cup almond milk
- 1 tablespoon honey
- 1 scoop vanilla protein powder

Preparation:

1. Pit the cherries if needed.
2. Combine all ingredients in a blender.
3. Blend until well combined.
4. Pour into a glass and savor the cherry-almond goodness!

Prep Time: 5 minutes

9. Blueberry-Banana Smoothie

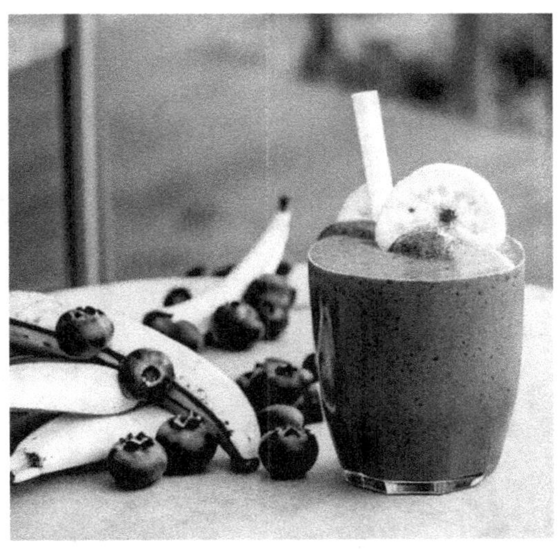

Ingredients:

- 1 cup frozen blueberries
- 1 ripe banana
- 1 cup whole milk
- 1 tablespoon honey
- 1/4 cup walnuts

Preparation:

1. Peel and chop the banana.

2. Combine all ingredients in a blender.

3. Blend until smooth and creamy.

4. Pour into a glass and enjoy the antioxidant-rich smoothie!

Prep Time: 5 minutes

10. Creamy Pineapple-Coconut Burst

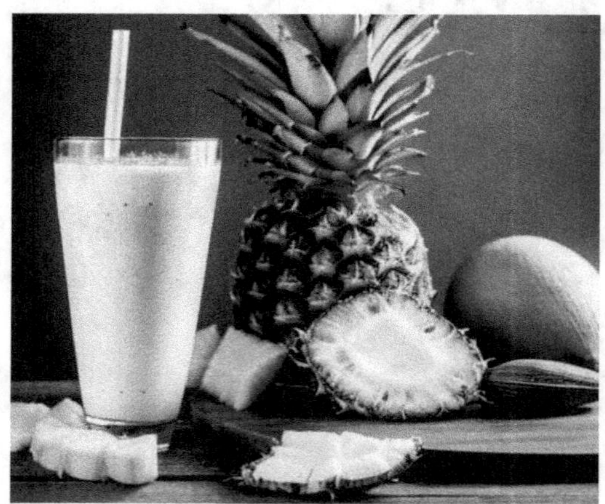

Ingredients:

- 1 cup frozen pineapple chunks
- 1/2 cup canned coconut milk
- 1 cup coconut water
- 1 tablespoon chia seeds

- 1 tablespoon shredded coconut

Preparation:
1. Combine all ingredients in a blender.
2. Blend until creamy and well mixed.
3. Pour into a glass and imagine yourself in a tropical paradise!

Prep Time: 5 minutes

11. Green Apple-Oatmeal Energizer

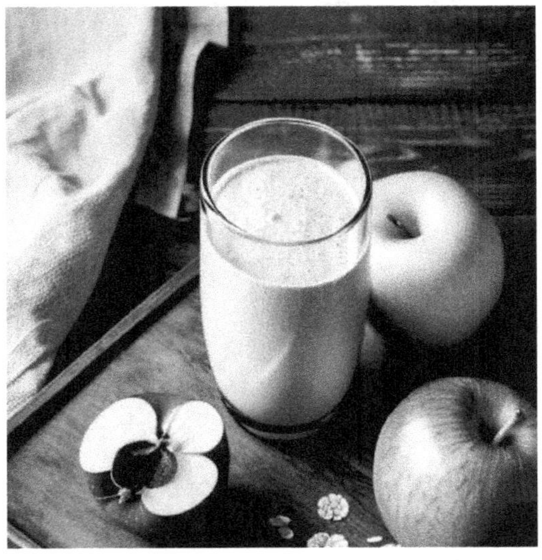

Ingredients:

- 1 green apple, cored and chopped
- 1/4 cup almond butter
- 1 cup almond milk
- 1/4 cup rolled oats
- 1 tablespoon honey
- 1/2 teaspoon ground cinnamon

Preparation:

1. Core and chop the green apple.

2. Combine all ingredients in a blender.

3. Blend until smooth and creamy.

4. Pour into a glass and enjoy the apple-cinnamon goodness!

Prep Time: 5 minutes

12. Peanut Butter-Banana Protein Boost

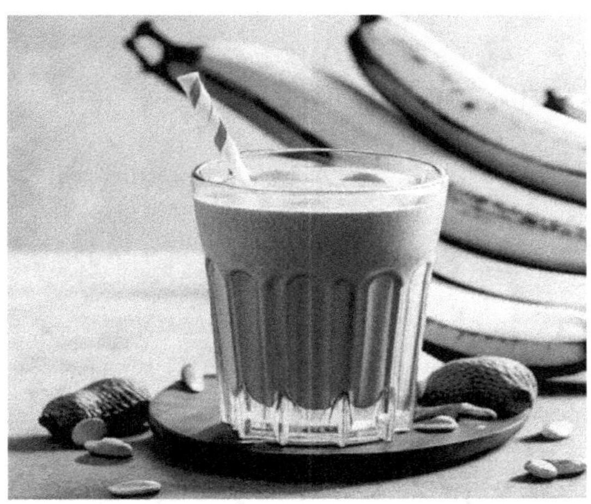

Ingredients:

- 2 ripe bananas utter
- 2 tablespoons natural peanut butter
- 1 cup whole milk
- 1 scoop chocolate protein powder
- 1 tablespoon honey
- 1/4 cup peanuts (optional: roasted for extra flavor)

Preparation:

1. Peel and chop the bananas.
2. Combine all ingredients in a blender.

3. Blend until well mixed.

4. Pour into a glass and indulge in the peanut-buttery delight!

Prep Time: 5 minutes

13. Mixed Berry-Spinach Vitality

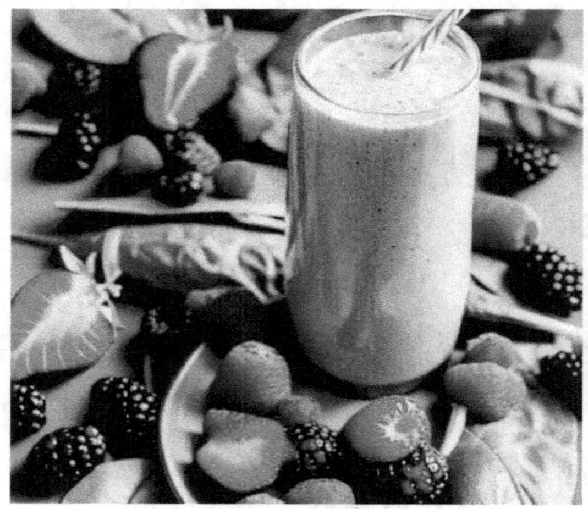

Ingredients:

- 1 cup berries(strawberries, blueberries and raspberries)
- 1 cup fresh spinach leaves
- 1/2 cup Greek yogurt
- 1 tablespoon honey

- 1/2 cup water or coconut water

Preparation:

1. Wash the spinach leaves thoroughly.
2. Combine all ingredients in a blender.
3. Blend until smooth and creamy.
4. Pour into a glass and enjoy the nutritious berry-spinach combo!

Prep Time: 5 minutes

14. Mocha-Banana Protein Delight

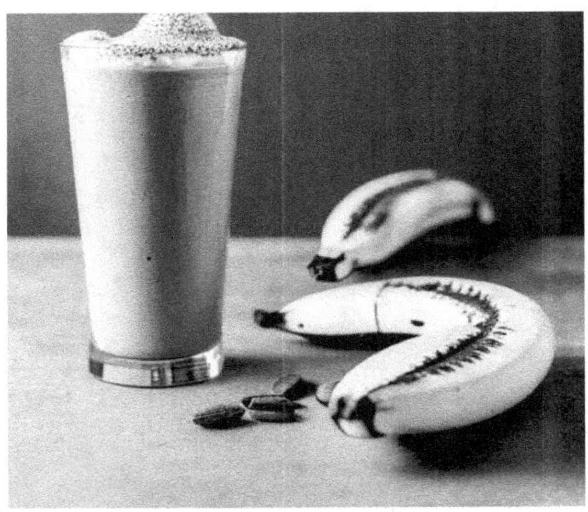

Ingredients:

- 1 ripe banana
- 1 tablespoon almond butter
- 1 cup cold coffee
- 1 scoop chocolate protein powder
- 1 tablespoon honey
- 1/4 cup oats

Preparation:

1. Peel and chop the banana.
2. Combine all ingredients in a blender.
3. Blend until creamy and frothy.
4. Pour into a glass and relish the mocha flavor!

Prep Time: 5 minutes

15. Raspberry-Chia Bliss

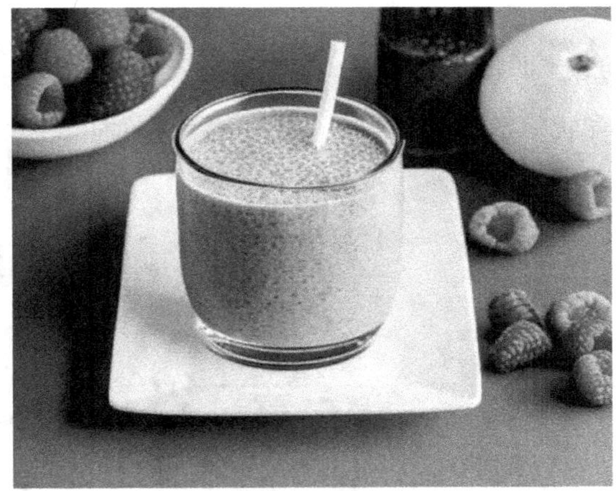

Ingredients:

- 1 cup frozen raspberries
- 1 tablespoon chia seeds
- 1 cup almond milk
- 1 tablespoon honey
- 1/4 cup cashews

Preparation:

1. Combine all ingredients in a blender.

2. Blend until smooth and creamy.

3. Pour into a glass and savor the raspberry goodness!

16. Vanilla-Date Almond Power

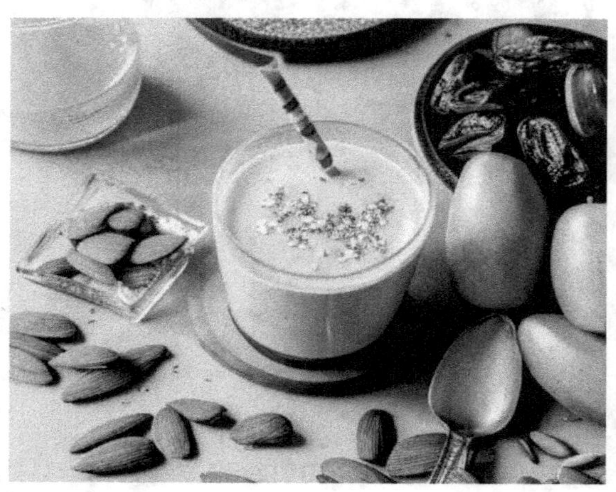

Ingredients:

- 2 ripe bananas
- 4 Medjool dates, pitted
- 1 cup whole milk
- 1 teaspoon vanilla extract
- 1/4 cup almonds

Preparation:

1. Peel and chop the bananas.
2. Combine all ingredients in a blender.
3. Blend until creamy and smooth.

4. Pour into a glass and enjoy the sweetness of dates!

Prep Time: 5 minutes

17. Mango-Coconut Chia Boost

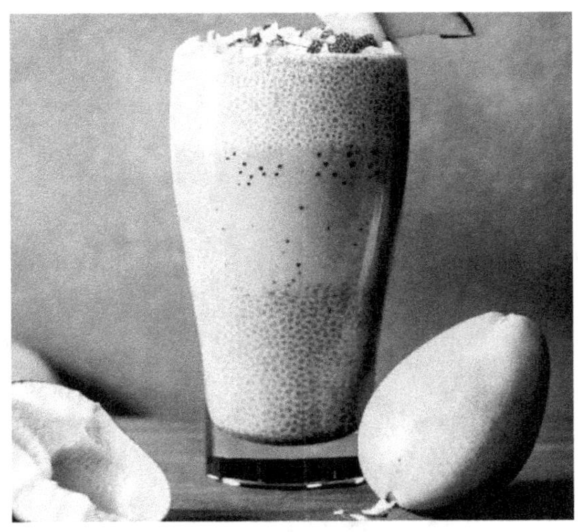

Ingredients:
- 1 cup frozen mango chunks
- 1/2 cup canned coconut milk
- 1 tablespoon chia seeds
- 1 tablespoon honey
- 1/4 cup toasted coconut flakes

Preparation:

1. Combine all ingredients in a blender.
2. Blend until creamy and well mixed.
3. Pour into a glass and enjoy the tropical fusion!

Prep Time: 5 minutes

18. Triple Berry-Protein Punch

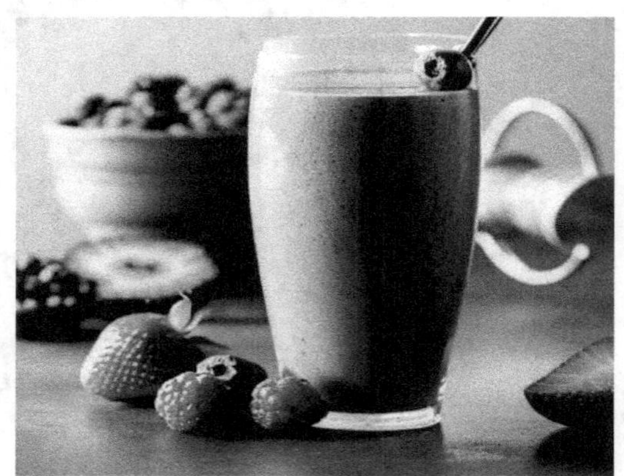

Ingredients:

- 1 cup mixed berries (strawberries, blueberries, blackberries)
- 1/4 cup Greek yogurt
- 1 cup almond milk

- 1 scoop vanilla protein powder
- 1 tablespoon honey

Preparation:

1. Wash the berries and remove stems.
2. Combine all ingredients in a blender.
3. Blend until smooth and creamy.
4. Pour into a glass and enjoy the protein-packed goodness!

Prep Time: 5 minutes

19. Peanut Butter-Chocolate Banana Bliss

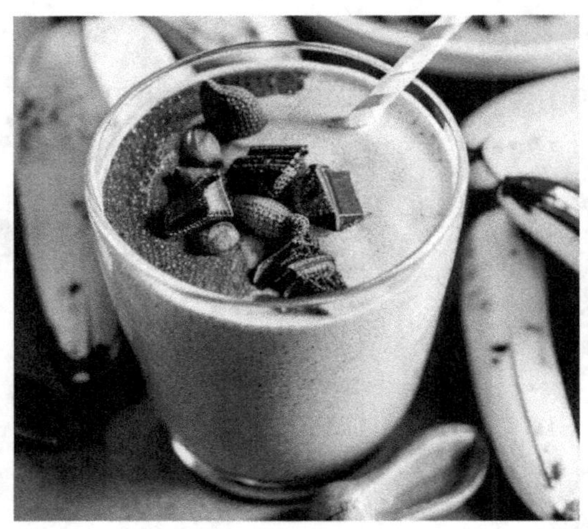

Ingredients:

- 1 ripe banana
- 2 tablespoons natural peanut butter
- 1 cup chocolate almond milk
- 1 tablespoon cocoa powder
- 1 tablespoon honey
- 1/4 cup granola

Preparation:

1. Peel and chop the banana.
2. Combine all ingredients in a blender.

3. Blend until smooth and creamy.

4. Pour into a glass and indulge in the peanut-buttery chocolate delight!

Prep Time: 5 minutes

20. Spinach-Mango Coconut Delight

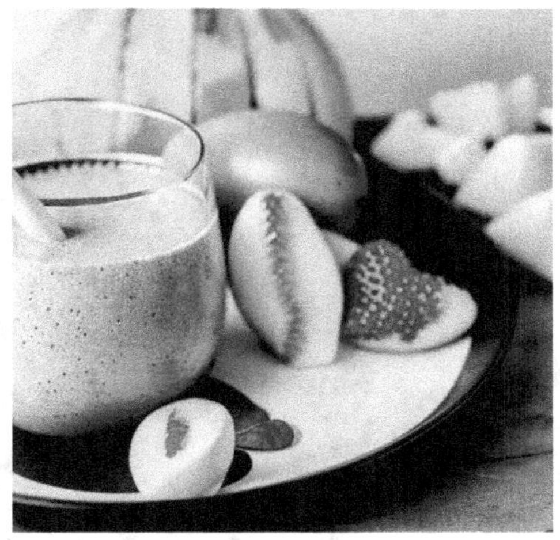

Ingredients:

- 1 cup fresh spinach leaves
- 1 cup frozen mango chunks
- 1/2 cup canned coconut milk
- 1 tablespoon honey
- 1/2 cup water or coconut water

Preparation:

1. Wash the spinach leaves thoroughly.
2. Combine all ingredients in a blender.
3. Blend until smooth and creamy.
4. Pour into a glass and enjoy the green tropical fusion!

Prep Time: 5 minutes

21. Cherry-Almond Oat Blast

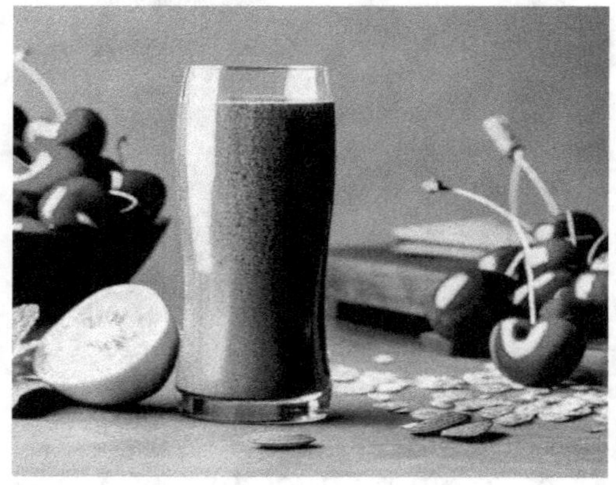

Ingredients:

- 1 cup frozen cherries
- 1/4 cup almond butter

- 1 cup almond milk
- 1 tablespoon honey
- 1/4 cup rolled oats

Preparation:
1. Pit the cherries if needed.
2. Combine all ingredients in a blender.
3. Blend until well combined.
4. Pour into a glass and savor the cherry-almond oat goodness!

Prep Time: 5 minutes

22. Blueberry-Banana Nutty Delight

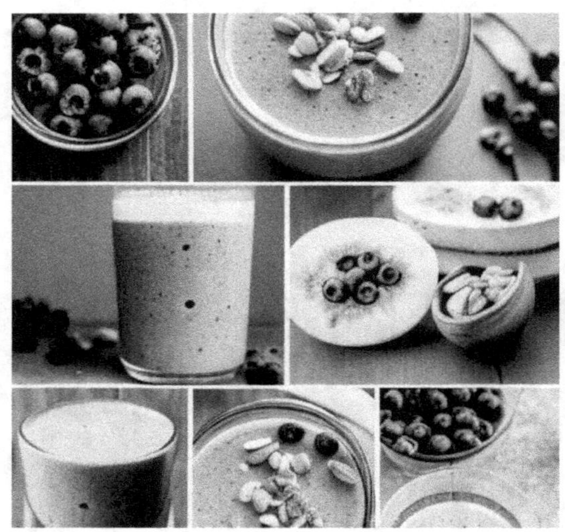

Ingredients:

- 1 cup frozen blueberries
- 1 ripe banana
- 1 cup whole milk
- 1 tablespoon honey
- 1/4 cup mixed nuts (almonds, walnuts, cashews)

Preparation:

1. Peel and chop the banana.
2. Combine all ingredients in a blender.
3. Blend until smooth and creamy.

4. Pour into a glass and enjoy the nutty berry combo!

Prep Time: 5 minutes

23. Creamy Pineapple-Mango Burst

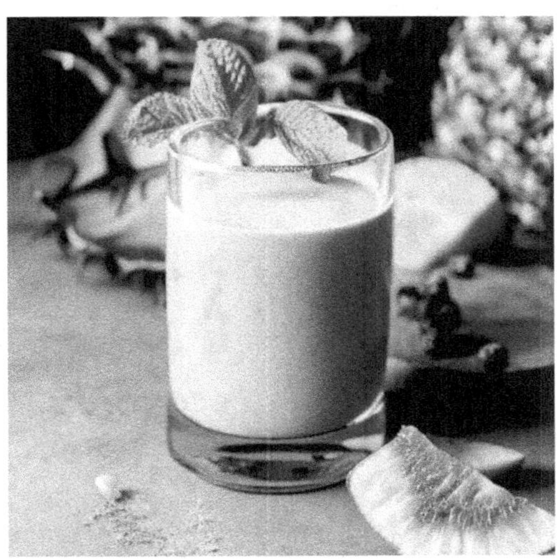

Ingredients:
- 1 cup frozen pineapple chunks
- 1 cup frozen mango chunks
- 1 cup coconut water
- 1 tablespoon honey
- 1/4 cup Greek yogurt

Preparation:
1. Combine all ingredients in a blender.
2. Blend until creamy and well mixed.
3. Pour into a glass and experience the tropical mango-pineapple delight!

Prep Time: 5 minutes

24. Green Kiwi-Banana Boost

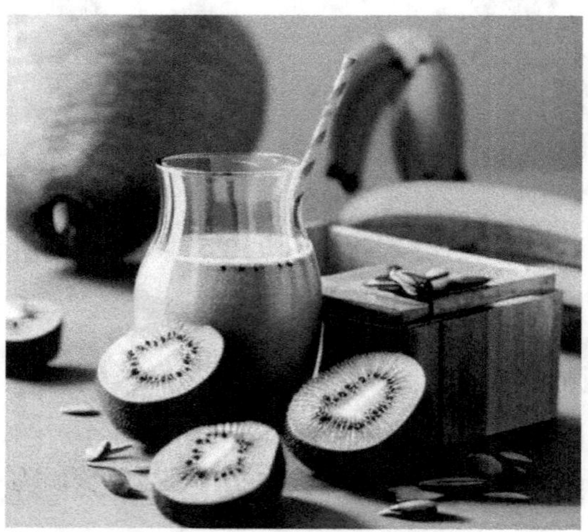

Ingredients:
- 2 ripe kiwis, peeled
- 1 ripe banana

- 1 cup spinach leaves
- 1 cup almond milk
- 1 tablespoon honey

Preparation:
1. Peel and chop the kiwis and banana.
2. Wash the spinach leaves thoroughly.
3. Combine all ingredients in a blender.
4. Blend until smooth and creamy.
5. Pour into a glass and enjoy the vitamin-packed green smoothie!

Prep Time: 5 minutes

25. Peanut Butter-Oatmeal Protein Punch

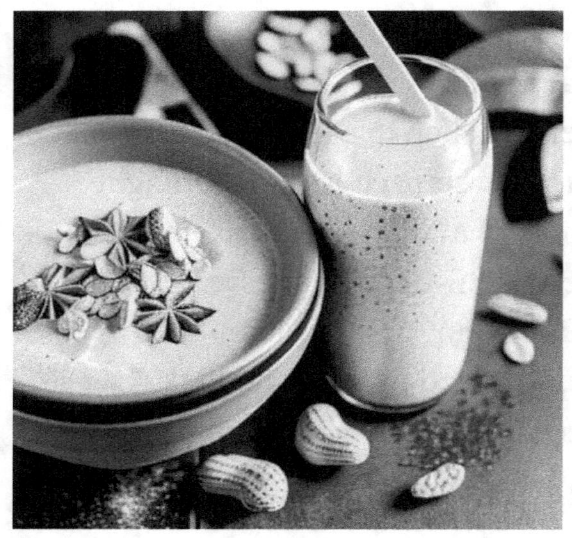

Ingredients:

- 2 tablespoons natural peanut butter
- 1/4 cup rolled oats
- 1 cup whole milk
- 1 scoop vanilla protein powder
- 1 tablespoon honey
- 1/4 teaspoon ground nutmeg

Preparation:

1. Combine all ingredients in a blender.

2. Blend until smooth and creamy.

3. Pour into a glass and savor the peanut butter-oat goodness!

Prep Time: 5 minutes

26. Raspberry-Coconut Protein Blast

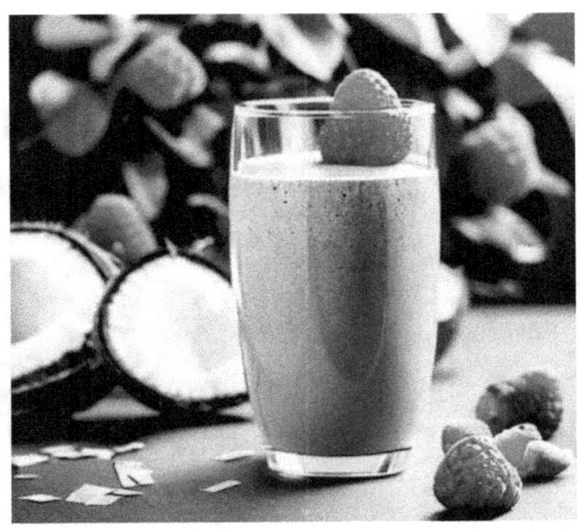

Ingredients:

- 1 cup frozen raspberries
- 1/2 cup canned coconut milk
- 1 scoop vanilla protein powder
- 1 tablespoon honey
- 1/4 cup shredded coconut

Preparation:

1. Combine all ingredients in a blender.
2. Blend until creamy and well mixed.
3. Pour into a glass and enjoy the berry-coconut fusion!

Prep Time: 5 minutes

27. Chocolate-Banana Nut Powerhouse

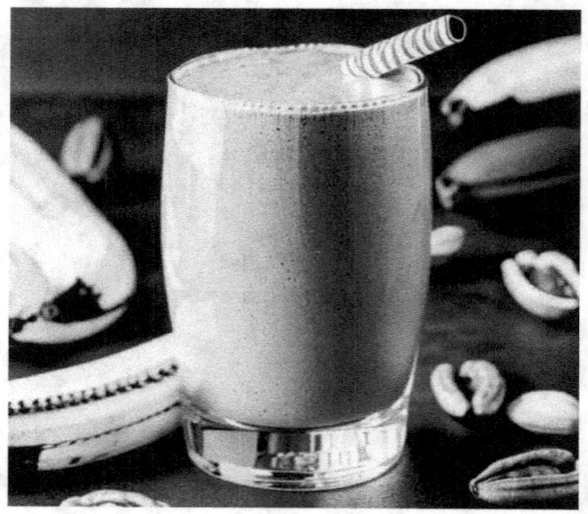

Ingredients:

- 1 ripe banana
- 2 tablespoons almond butter

- 1 cup chocolate almond milk
- 1 tablespoon cocoa powder
- 1 tablespoon honey
- 1/4 cup mixed nuts (almonds, walnuts, cashews)

Preparation:

1. Peel and chop the banana.
2. Combine all ingredients in a blender.
3. Blend until smooth and creamy.
4. Pour into a glass and indulge in the chocolate-nutty delight!

Prep Time: 5 minutes

28. Mango-Coconut Spinach Kick

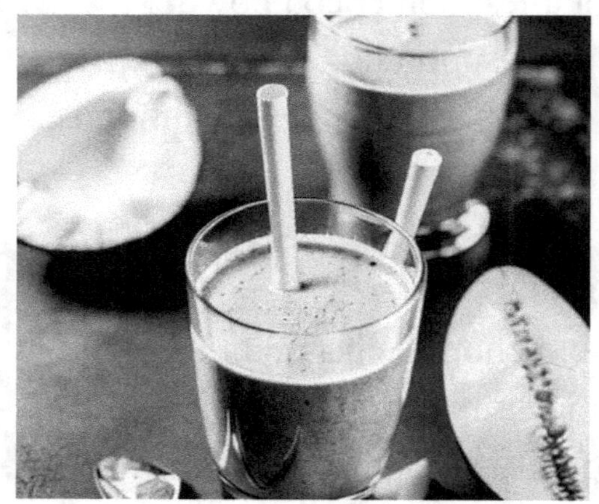

Ingredients:

- 1 cup frozen mango chunks
- 1/2 cup canned coconut milk
- 1 cup fresh spinach leaves
- 1 tablespoon honey
- 1/2 cup water or coconut water

Preparation:

1. Wash the spinach leaves thoroughly.
2. Combine all ingredients in a blender.
3. Blend until smooth and creamy.
4. Pour into a glass and enjoy the green tropical kick!

Prep Time: 5 minutes

29. Mixed Berry-Date Energizer

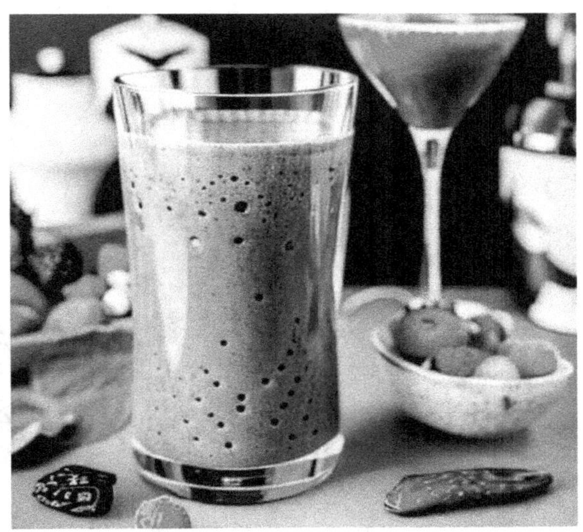

Ingredients:

- 1 cup mixed berries (strawberries, blueberries, raspberries)
- 4 Medjool dates, pitted
- 1 cup almond milk
- 1 tablespoon honey
- 1/4 cup almonds

Preparation:

1. Wash the berries and remove stems.

2. Combine all ingredients in a blender.

3. Blend until smooth and creamy.

4. Pour into a glass and enjoy the berry-date goodness!

Prep Time: 5 minutes

30. Vanilla-Almond Power Punch

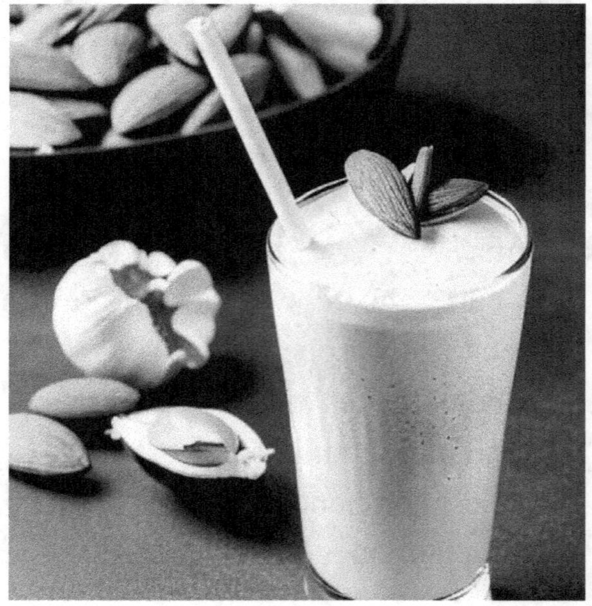

Ingredients:

- 1 cup whole milk
- 1/4 cup almonds
- 1 teaspoon vanilla extract
- 1 tablespoon honey
- 1/4 cup oats

Preparation:

1. Combine all ingredients in a blender.

2. Blend until smooth and creamy.

3. Pour into a glass and savor the vanilla-almond goodness!

Prep Time: 5 minutes

Enjoy your delicious and nutritious weight gain smoothies! Remember to customize these recipes based on your preferences and dietary needs. Happy blending!

Conclusion

The journey we've embarked upon together in this smoothie for weight gain book has been nothing short of transformative. We have explored the delightful world of nutritious and delicious smoothies, crafted specifically to help you reach your weight gain goals while nourishing your body from within.

As we bid farewell, remember that gaining weight healthily is not just about adding empty calories or mindlessly indulging in sugary treats. It is about embracing a holistic approach that prioritizes the right nutrients, healthy fats, proteins, and fiber to support your body's needs and enhance your overall well-being.

Each smoothie recipe shared within these pages is more than just a blend of ingredients; it is a symbol of empowerment and self-care. It's about finding joy in the process of nourishing yourself and celebrating the changes you'll witness along the way.

So, savor each sip, relish every moment of this journey, and know that you have the knowledge and power to achieve your weight gain goals. As you continue to blend these smoothies into your daily routine, may you find strength in your newfound confidence, and may your body flourish with vitality and energy.

Always remember, your body is a temple, and every smoothie you create is a testament to your dedication to loving and caring for it. Embrace your uniqueness, trust in the process, and let these smoothies be the catalyst for your transformation.

Now, go forth with a heart full of determination and a blender full of endless possibilities. The power to shape your destiny and embrace the healthiest version of yourself lies within each velvety smooth sip. Here's to a vibrant and fulfilling life filled with the joy of self-discovery and the delight of savoring your journey to newfound strength and happiness.

Cheers to you and your magnificent transformation!

www.ingramcontent.com/pod-product-compliance
Lightning Source LLC
Chambersburg PA
CBHW070734260726
48660CB00007B/2835